COMPLETE GUIDE TO

MENISCUS REPAIR SURGERY

Essential Handbook To Effective Treatments, Recovery Strategies, and Expert Insights for Knee Injury Relief

DR. BRUNO HORAN

Disclaimer:

The information provided in this book, is intended for general informational purposes only and should not be considered as professional advice.

The author has made every effort to ensure the accuracy of the information presented. However, readers are advised to consult with a qualified healthcare professional before attempting any herbal remedies or making significant changes to their wellness routine. Individual health conditions vary, and what may be suitable for one person may not be appropriate for another.

It is important to note that the author is not in any endorsement deal, partnership, or affiliation with any organization, brand, or company mentioned in this book. Any references to specific products or services are based on the author's personal experience or general knowledge and do not imply an endorsement or promotion of those products or services

Contents

ABOUT THIS BOOK

In the intricate realm of knee health, understanding the pivotal role of the meniscus is paramount. Situated between the femur and tibia, the meniscus serves as a crucial shock absorber and stabilizer, essential for maintaining knee functionality and overall joint integrity. This book, Meniscus Repair Surgery, delves deep into the nuances of meniscal injuries, offering comprehensive insights that empower readers to navigate their treatment journey with confidence and clarity.

From the onset, the book elucidates the anatomical intricacies of the knee and expounds upon the specific functions of the meniscus. It meticulously outlines various types of meniscal tears, from radial to complex, and meticulously details the telltale signs and symptoms indicative of a torn meniscus. Through detailed descriptions and diagnostic approaches encompassing physical examinations and advanced imaging techniques, the book underscores the criticality of timely diagnosis and intervention in mitigating long-term complications.

Beyond the diagnostic phase, Meniscus Repair Surgery meticulously explores both non-surgical and surgical treatment avenues. It delves into the efficacy of conservative approaches such as RICE therapy, physical rehabilitation, and pharmacological management, while candidly addressing their limitations. Emphasizing the surgical realm, the book offers a comprehensive panorama of meniscus repair surgeries, distinguishing between meniscectomy and repair procedures. It elucidates the nuances of arthroscopic surgery, unveiling its procedural intricacies, post-operative rehabilitation protocols, and associated risks.

Throughout its narrative, Meniscus Repair Surgery champions a holistic approach to patient care, encompassing pre-operative preparations, anesthesia considerations, and the pivotal role of mental readiness in fostering positive surgical outcomes. It elucidates the day-of-surgery dynamics, demystifying procedural steps and highlighting the collaborative efforts of the surgical team.

Post-operative chapters meticulously guide readers through the intricacies of recovery, offering pragmatic strategies for pain management, structured physical therapy regimens, and proactive measures to monitor progress. Addressing common concerns and potential complications with clarity, the book equips readers with the knowledge needed to navigate the recovery phase with resilience and informed decision-making.

Anchoring its narrative in real-life experiences, Meniscus Repair Surgery amplifies patient voices through compelling anecdotes and firsthand accounts. These narratives offer invaluable insights into the challenges and triumphs associated with meniscal repair, fostering a sense of community and solidarity among readers facing similar journeys.

Lastly, the book anticipates and addresses reader inquiries through a robust FAQ section, covering topics ranging from recovery timelines and post-surgical aids to preventive measures and long-term prognosis. By preemptively addressing these concerns, Meniscus Repair Surgery serves as an indispensable companion, empowering readers with the knowledge and confidence to navigate their meniscal injury journey effectively.

CHAPTER ONE

UNDERSTANDING THE MENISCUS

The knee joint is crucial for mobility and stability, composed of bones, ligaments, tendons, and the menisci.

The meniscus, consisting of two C-shaped pieces of cartilage, serves as a cushion between the thigh bone (femur) and the shin bone (tibia).

These structures play a pivotal role in distributing weight, absorbing shock, and enhancing joint stability during movements such as walking, running, and jumping.

Anatomy Of The Knee And The Role Of The Meniscus

The knee joint is a hinge joint formed by the femur, tibia, and patella (kneecap), surrounded by various ligaments and muscles that enable flexibility and strength.

The menisci are positioned between the femur and tibia, with the medial (inner) and lateral (outer) menisci absorbing forces and providing stability. Their crescent shape adapts to changes in joint shape during movement, optimizing contact and distributing load evenly across the joint surface.

Types Of Meniscus Tears: Radial, Horizontal, Complex

Meniscus tears can vary in type and severity, commonly classified into radial, horizontal, and complex tears. Radial tears extend from the inner to the outer edge of the meniscus, potentially disrupting its ability to function effectively.

Horizontal tears occur parallel to the meniscus's surface and may compromise its stability. Complex tears involve a combination of both radial and horizontal components, often requiring careful assessment and treatment tailored to the tear's characteristics.

Symptoms And Signs Of A Torn Meniscus

Symptoms of a torn meniscus often include pain, swelling, stiffness, and a sensation of locking or catching within the knee joint. Patients may experience difficulty straightening or bending the knee fully, coupled with instability during weight-bearing activities. Signs such as localized tenderness along the joint line and positive physical examination maneuvers, like McMurray's test, aid in diagnosing the presence and extent of a meniscus tear.

Diagnosis Through Physical Examination And Imaging Techniques

Diagnosing a torn meniscus typically begins with a thorough physical examination, assessing range of motion, joint stability, and specific maneuvers to elicit pain or mechanical symptoms. Imaging techniques such as magnetic resonance imaging (MRI) provide detailed visualization of the menisci and surrounding structures, helping to confirm the diagnosis, assess tear size and location, and guide treatment decisions.

Importance Of Timely Treatment

Timely treatment of a torn meniscus is essential to prevent further damage, alleviate symptoms, and restore knee function. Early intervention can often preserve the meniscus's integrity and reduce the risk of complications such as joint degeneration or secondary injuries. Treatment strategies may include conservative measures like rest, ice, compression, and physical therapy, or in some cases, surgical repair or partial meniscectomy, depending on the tear's severity and the patient's factors.

This structured approach aims to provide clarity on the anatomy, types of tears, symptoms, diagnosis, and the critical importance of timely intervention in managing a torn meniscus effectively.

CHAPTER TWO

NON-SURGICAL TREATMENTS

Rest, Ice, Compression, And Elevation (RICE) Therapy

Resting the affected knee is crucial in the initial stages of treating meniscus injuries. This helps reduce strain on the injured area and promotes natural healing.

Applying ice intermittently helps to decrease swelling and alleviate pain by constricting blood vessels. Compression, through the use of an elastic bandage or brace, provides support and further reduces swelling.

Elevating the leg above heart level also aids in minimizing swelling and enhancing blood flow back to the heart.

Physical Therapy And Strengthening Exercises

Physical therapy plays a pivotal role in rehabilitating meniscus injuries, aiming to restore strength, flexibility, and functionality to the knee.

A physical therapist designs exercises tailored to the individual's injury severity and recovery stage. Initially, exercises focus on regaining range of motion and reducing stiffness.

As recovery progresses, strengthening exercises target the muscles surrounding the knee, such as the quadriceps and hamstrings, to provide better support and stability.

Medications For Pain And Inflammation Management

Nonsteroidal anti-inflammatory drugs (NSAIDs) are commonly prescribed to alleviate pain and reduce inflammation associated with meniscus injuries.

These medications, such as ibuprofen or naproxen, help manage discomfort and enable individuals to participate more comfortably in physical therapy and daily activities.

In some cases, acetaminophen may be recommended for pain relief if NSAIDs are not suitable due to individual health factors.

Limitations And Considerations For Non-Surgical Approaches

While non-surgical treatments like RICE therapy, physical therapy, and medications can effectively manage many meniscus injuries, they may have limitations.

Some tears, particularly larger or complex tears, may not respond adequately to conservative treatments alone. Factors such as the tear's location, size, and the patient's overall health and activity level influence the treatment approach.

When Non-Surgical Methods May Not Be Sufficient

Non-surgical methods may not suffice for certain meniscus injuries, especially if symptoms persist or worsen despite conservative treatments. Factors indicating the need for surgical intervention include significant pain that limits daily activities, mechanical symptoms like catching or locking of the knee, or inability to bear weight on the affected leg. Surgical consultation may be recommended to address the tear more directly and prevent long-term complications.

CHAPTER THREE

SURGICAL OPTIONS

Types Of Meniscus Repair Surgeries: Meniscectomy Vs. Meniscus Repair

When faced with a meniscus injury, understanding the surgical options is crucial. Meniscus surgeries primarily fall into two categories: meniscectomy and meniscus repair.

Meniscectomy involves removing the damaged part of the meniscus. This procedure is often chosen when the tear is in the outer edge of the meniscus where blood supply is adequate for healing. It's a quicker procedure with shorter recovery times compared to repair.

Meniscus Repair, on the other hand, aims to preserve the meniscus. It involves stitching the torn edges together or reattaching the meniscus using sutures or anchors. This approach is preferred for tears in the inner part of the meniscus where blood supply is limited. Repair aims to restore the cushioning and stability provided by the meniscus, potentially preventing long-term joint issues.

Arthroscopic Surgery: Procedure And Benefits

Arthroscopic Surgery is the standard approach for both meniscectomy and meniscus repair due to its minimally invasive nature and precise outcomes. During arthroscopy, a small camera (arthroscope) is inserted through tiny incisions into the knee joint. This allows the surgeon to visualize the interior structures of the knee on a screen in real time.

The procedure begins with the surgeon making small incisions around the knee joint. The arthroscope, equipped with a light and camera, is then inserted to assess the meniscus tear. Small surgical instruments are used to perform the necessary repairs or removals.

Rehabilitation Timeline Post-Surgery

Rehabilitation after meniscus surgery is crucial for a successful recovery. The timeline varies depending on the type of surgery and individual factors, but generally follows a structured approach:

Immediately Post-Surgery: Patients may begin with gentle movement exercises to prevent stiffness and improve circulation.

First Few Weeks: Physical therapy starts, focusing on restoring the knee's range of motion and strengthening the surrounding muscles.

Weeks 4-12: As healing progresses, exercises become more challenging to regain full strength and stability.

Months 3-6: Return to normal activities, with continued focus on strengthening and flexibility.

Risks and Complications Associated with Surgery

While meniscus surgeries are generally safe, there are risks and potential complications to be aware of:

Infection: Although rare, any surgery carries a risk of infection. Proper sterile techniques and antibiotics help minimize this risk.

Blood Clots: Deep vein thrombosis (DVT) can occur, especially if immobility persists post-surgery. Compression stockings and early mobilization help prevent this.

Failure to Heal: In some cases, repaired menisci may not heal completely, leading to persistent symptoms or the need for further surgery.

Success Rates And Long-Term Outcomes

Success Rates: The success of meniscus surgery varies based on factors such as tear type, surgical technique, and patient age. Generally, meniscus repair shows higher success rates in younger patients with tears in the vascular zone of the meniscus.

Long-Term Outcomes: Patients often experience reduced pain and improved knee function after successful surgery. Long-term outcomes are favorable when rehabilitation protocols are followed diligently, promoting optimal healing and joint function restoration.

These insights into surgical options, procedures, rehabilitation, risks, and outcomes aim to empower patients with the knowledge to make informed decisions and facilitate a smoother recovery journey post-meniscus surgery.

CHAPTER FOUR

PREPARATION FOR SURGERY

Pre-Operative Consultations And Evaluations

Before undergoing meniscus repair surgery, several consultations and evaluations are essential to ensure you're well-prepared for the procedure.

Your orthopedic surgeon will conduct a thorough assessment of your knee joint to determine the extent of the meniscus damage and the most appropriate surgical approach.

This evaluation may include physical examinations, imaging tests such as MRI scans, and discussions about your medical history and any previous knee injuries or surgeries.

Steps To Prepare Your Home And Support System

Preparing your home environment and support system is crucial for a smooth recovery after meniscus repair surgery. Arrange for someone to accompany you on the day of surgery and assist you during the initial days of recovery.

Make sure your home is conducive to recovery by setting up a comfortable space where you can rest, placing essential items within easy reach, and ensuring clear pathways to avoid tripping hazards.

Understanding Anesthesia Options

Anesthesia plays a vital role in ensuring your comfort and safety during meniscus repair surgery. Your anesthesiologist will discuss the anesthesia options available, which may include general anesthesia or regional anesthesia techniques such as spinal or epidural anesthesia.

Understanding these options involves weighing factors such as your medical history, preferences, and the specific requirements of the surgical procedure.

Financial Considerations And Insurance Coverage

Navigating the financial aspects of meniscus repair surgery involves understanding costs, insurance coverage, and any out-of-pocket expenses you may incur.

Before surgery, discuss financial matters with your healthcare provider or surgical center to clarify payment methods, insurance billing processes, and potential costs associated with anesthesia, hospital stays, and post-operative care.

Mental Preparation And Managing Expectations

Preparing mentally for meniscus repair surgery involves managing expectations and understanding the recovery process. Discuss with your healthcare team what to expect before, during, and after surgery, including potential risks and complications. Engage in relaxation techniques, such as deep breathing or meditation, to reduce pre-surgery anxiety and promote a positive mindset towards your recovery journey.

CHAPTER FIVE

DAY OF SURGERY

What To Expect Upon Arrival At The Surgical Center

On the day of your meniscus repair surgery, you'll typically arrive at the surgical center early in the morning.

Upon arrival, you'll be greeted by the reception staff who will guide you through the check-in process. You'll be asked to provide identification and insurance information if you haven't already done so. After completing any necessary paperwork, a nurse or surgical assistant will escort you to a pre-operative area where you'll change into a surgical gown.

Pre-Operative Procedures And Preparations

Before surgery begins, several important pre-operative procedures will take place to ensure your safety and readiness for the procedure. You'll meet with your anesthesiologist who will review your medical history, discuss anesthesia options, and address any concerns you may have.

Vital signs such as blood pressure, heart rate, and temperature will be measured, and an IV line will be started to administer fluids and medications during and after surgery.

Overview Of The Surgical Team And Their Roles

The surgical team consists of several key members, each with specific roles to ensure the success of your procedure.

The surgeon will lead the operation, assisted by surgical nurses and technicians who will provide support throughout. The anesthesiologist will monitor your vital signs and anesthesia levels during the surgery, adjusting as necessary to keep you comfortable and safe.

The Steps Of The Surgical Procedure Are Explained.

The meniscus repair surgery typically begins with the administration of anesthesia, either general anesthesia where you are unconscious throughout the procedure, or regional anesthesia where only the lower part of your body is numbed.

Once you are sedated, the surgical team will clean and sterilize the surgical site before making small incisions around the knee joint. Using specialized instruments and a small camera called an arthroscope, the surgeon will locate and assess the damaged meniscus tissue.

Post-Surgery Recovery Room And Initial Recovery Process

After the surgery is completed, you'll be moved to a recovery room where you'll awaken from anesthesia under the care of experienced nurses. Your vital signs will be monitored closely, and pain management will be addressed promptly to ensure your comfort.

The surgical team will provide instructions for post-operative care, including when and how to start gentle exercises and what to expect in terms of swelling and discomfort in the initial hours and days following surgery.

CHAPTER SIX

POST-OPERATIVE CARE

After meniscus repair surgery, proper post-operative care is crucial for a successful recovery. This phase begins immediately after surgery and continues through the rehabilitation process. Here's what you need to know to ensure a smooth recovery:

Immediate Post-Surgery Care Instructions

Following surgery, you will be monitored closely in the recovery room until you are stable. You may experience some pain and discomfort, which is normal.

Ice packs and elevation of the leg can help reduce swelling. Your healthcare team will provide instructions on how to care for the surgical site and manage any initial discomfort.

Pain Management Strategies And Medications

Pain management is an important part of your recovery. Your doctor will prescribe medications to help control pain. It's important to take these medications as directed to stay ahead of any discomfort. Additionally, applying ice packs and keeping the leg elevated can help reduce pain and swelling.

Physical Therapy Exercises And Rehabilitation Program

Physical therapy plays a critical role in restoring strength and function to your knee after meniscus repair surgery.

Your physical therapist will design a personalized rehabilitation program tailored to your specific needs. Initially, you may focus on gentle range-of-motion exercises and gradually progress to strengthening exercises as your knee heals.

Activities To Avoid During Recovery

During the initial phase of recovery, it's important to avoid activities that could stress or damage your healing knee.

These may include high-impact sports, running, jumping, and twisting motions. Your doctor will provide specific guidelines based on your surgery and individual progress.

Monitoring Progress And Follow-Up Appointments

Regular follow-up appointments with your surgeon are essential to monitor your progress and adjust your recovery plan as needed.

Your doctor will assess your healing, check for any complications, and guide you on when it's safe to gradually resume normal activities.

Be sure to attend all scheduled appointments and communicate any concerns or changes in your recovery.

By following these post-operative care instructions, participating actively in your rehabilitation program, and staying in close communication with your healthcare team, you can optimize your recovery and return to your daily activities with confidence.

CHAPTER SEVEN

COMMON CONCERNS AND COMPLICATIONS

During the recovery from meniscus repair surgery, several common concerns and potential complications may arise, requiring attention and proper management.

Infection Prevention And Wound Care

One of the primary concerns post-surgery is preventing infection and ensuring proper wound care. Your surgeon will provide specific instructions on how to care for your surgical site.

This typically involves keeping the incision clean and dry, and possibly applying an antibiotic ointment as directed.

It's crucial to monitor for signs of infection such as increased redness, warmth, swelling, or drainage from the incision site.

If you notice any of these symptoms, it's essential to contact your surgeon promptly for further evaluation and treatment.

Managing Swelling And Bruising

Swelling and bruising around the knee are common after meniscus repair surgery. To manage swelling effectively, your surgeon may recommend using ice packs and elevating your leg.

Ice can help reduce inflammation and alleviate discomfort. Additionally, gentle exercises and movements as instructed by your physical therapist can aid in improving circulation and reducing swelling over time. Bruising usually resolves on its own but can be managed with rest and elevation.

Signs Of Complications: When To Contact Your Surgeon

While complications are rare, it's essential to be aware of signs that may indicate a problem requiring medical attention. If you experience severe pain that is not relieved by prescribed pain medications, sudden onset of significant swelling, inability to bear weight on the affected leg, or any other unusual symptoms, contact your surgeon immediately. Prompt intervention can prevent complications and ensure optimal recovery.

Rehabilitation Setbacks And How To Address Them

Rehabilitation following meniscus repair surgery is a crucial part of recovery, but setbacks can occur. Common setbacks include stiffness, difficulty achieving full range of motion, or muscle weakness around the knee.

If you encounter these challenges, your physical therapist will adjust your rehabilitation program accordingly.

This may involve additional exercises, manual therapy techniques, or modifications to your activity level to promote gradual improvement.

Long-Term Impact On Knee Function And Activity Levels

Understanding the long-term impact of meniscus repair surgery on knee function and activity levels is important for setting realistic expectations.

Many patients experience significant improvement in knee function and can return to their previous level of activity after completing rehabilitation.

However, individual outcomes can vary based on factors such as the extent of the injury, surgical technique, and adherence to rehabilitation protocols.

Your surgeon and physical therapist will work closely with you to optimize your recovery and maximize your long-term outcomes.

By addressing these common concerns and being aware of potential complications, you can navigate your recovery from meniscus repair surgery with confidence.

Following your surgeon's recommendations, participating actively in rehabilitation, and promptly addressing any issues that arise will support your journey toward restored knee health and function.

CHAPTER EIGHT

PATIENT STORIES AND EXPERIENCES

Real-Life Accounts Of Meniscus Repair Surgeries

Patients undergoing meniscus repair surgeries often recount their journeys with a mix of apprehension, hope, and determination. Many describe the initial discomfort and uncertainty before surgery, where the prospect of returning to normal activities seemed distant.

However, as they progressed through treatment and rehabilitation, their narratives often pivot towards resilience and eventual triumph.

One patient, Sarah, recalls her experience vividly. "Before the surgery, I was worried about how long it would take to recover," she shares. "But the surgery went smoothly, and my doctor assured me that with proper care, I could regain mobility." Sarah's story underscores the importance of trust in medical advice and the gradual improvement that follows surgery.

Challenges Faced During Recovery And Rehabilitation

Recovery from meniscus repair surgery presents various challenges that patients navigate with determination. Pain management and restricted movement are common early hurdles.

"The first weeks were tough," reflects Mark, another patient. "I had to be patient with myself and follow the rehabilitation plan meticulously."

Mark's experience highlights the importance of adhering to post-operative care guidelines and the gradual return to physical activities.

For many patients, the mental challenge of staying motivated during rehabilitation can be as demanding as the physical aspects.

"There were times when I felt discouraged," admits Lisa. "But focusing on small milestones and celebrating each improvement helped me stay positive."

Lisa's journey reflects the emotional resilience required during recovery and the support network that plays a crucial role.

Success Stories And Return To Normal Activities

Success stories following meniscus repair surgeries are inspirational, showcasing the potential for full recovery and return to normal activities. John, an avid runner, shares his journey.

"I was worried I wouldn't be able to run again," he confides. "But with the right treatment and dedication to rehabilitation, I gradually resumed running."

John's success serves as motivation for others facing similar challenges, illustrating the possibilities after surgery.

Advice From Patients On Coping With Surgery

Patients often offer valuable advice based on their experiences with meniscus repair surgery. "Listen to your body," advises Rachel. "Rest when you need to and don't rush your recovery." Rachel's advice emphasizes self-awareness and patience during the healing process, crucial elements in achieving optimal outcomes.

Lessons Learned And Tips For Future Patients

Reflecting on their journeys, patients share lessons learned and practical tips for those about to undergo meniscus repair surgery.

"Prepare your home for post-operative comfort," suggests David. "Having essentials within reach reduces stress during recovery."

David's tip underscores the importance of proactive planning and creating a supportive environment for recuperation.

Each patient story and piece of advice contributes to a comprehensive understanding of meniscus repair surgery, offering insights that guide future patients through their recoveries.

These narratives underscore the resilience, determination, and optimism that define the journey toward healing and restored mobility.

CHAPTER NINE

FREQUENTLY ASKED QUESTIONS (FAQS)

How Long Does It Take To Recover From Meniscus Surgery?

Recovery time after meniscus surgery can vary depending on several factors, including the extent of the injury, the type of surgery performed, and individual healing rates.

Generally, patients can expect to begin weight-bearing and light activities within a few weeks after surgery. Full recovery, however, often takes several months. Physical therapy plays a crucial role in rehabilitation, helping to regain strength, flexibility, and normal joint function.

Your orthopedic surgeon will provide a personalized recovery timeline based on your specific case and progress during follow-up appointments.

Will I Need Crutches Or A Brace After Surgery?

The use of crutches or a brace post-surgery depends on the type of meniscus repair and your surgeon's recommendation. In cases where the meniscus is repaired rather than removed, crutches may be necessary initially to keep weight off the injured knee and allow healing. A knee brace might also be prescribed to provide support and stability as the knee regains strength. Your surgeon will assess your condition and prescribe the appropriate supportive devices to aid in your recovery.

Can A Meniscus Tear Heal On Its Own?

Unlike some tissues in the body, the meniscus has limited ability to heal on its own, especially in cases of significant tears or in the inner two-thirds where blood supply is poor.

However, small tears in the outer third of the meniscus, where there is a better blood supply, have a higher chance of healing without surgical intervention. Your orthopedic surgeon will evaluate the size, location, and type of tear to determine the most appropriate treatment plan, which may include non-surgical options such as rest, ice, physical therapy, and activity modification.

What Are The Chances Of The Tear Recurring?

The likelihood of a meniscus tear recurring after surgery depends on various factors, including the type of tear, the surgical technique used, post-operative rehabilitation, and adherence to activity modifications. In cases where the meniscus has been repaired, proper rehabilitation and avoiding high-impact activities during the recovery period are essential to minimize the risk of recurrence.

Your surgeon will provide specific guidelines on a gradual return to activities and strategies to reduce the chances of re-injury.

How Can I Prevent Future Meniscus Injuries?

Preventing future meniscus injuries involves maintaining good knee health through a combination of strength training, flexibility exercises, and proper body mechanics during physical activities. Strengthening the muscles around the knee, particularly the quadriceps and hamstrings, can help provide better support and stability to the joint. Avoiding sudden twisting or pivoting movements that place excessive stress on the knee can also reduce the risk of meniscus tears. If you participate in sports or activities that involve high-risk movements, wearing proper footwear and protective gear can provide additional support and minimize the likelihood of injury. Regularly engaging in low-impact exercises like swimming or cycling can also help maintain overall joint health and reduce the risk of future meniscus injuries.